THE BODY FACTOR

THE BODY FACTOR

The guide to get the maximum potential out of your body and live in fullness and harmony

The Wellness Factory

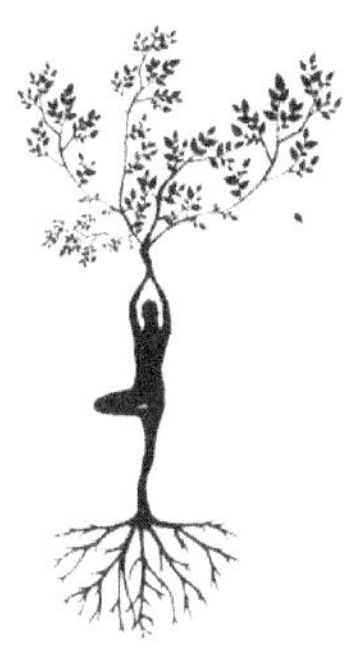

INTRODUCTORY WORDS 9

WE ARE DUAL BEINGS 13

EMOTIONAL WELL-BEING.......................................19

MAINTAINING LONG-TERM WELL-BEING 26

DISCOVER YOUR BODY 33

HEALTHY NUTRITION..48

DIET MYTHS 54

EXERCISE FOR WELLNESS..61

THE IMPORTANCE OF BUILDING MUSCLE......69

HOME FITNESS TRAINING 83

REST AND RELAXATION FOR WELLNESS.........92

FINAL WORDS 95

INTRODUCTORY WORDS

Some years ago, the media promoted the existence of an ideal body shape and insisted on the importance of making sacrifices to look like those models. The goal was not only difficult, but above all unrealistic, because those magazine models do not correspond to the genetic and cultural reality of most bodies. It was like pretending that with effort everyone could be two meters tall.

Nowadays, at least that ideal seems to have fallen a little behind, and aesthetic forms are promoted that are more in line with the prevailing variety. A specific weight and a particular body shape are no longer sold as the only possible ideal, so that everyone can conquer his or her own ideal.

The awareness that each body has its own potential opens up possibilities for everyone to adjust their way of life to get the best out of their own body. It is no longer only about universal measurements of weight, size, shapes... The expression in vogue today in terms of body and emotional care advises to be the best version of yourself. This is just because the ideal to look for is in us, it is not equated to that of others and is determined by our genes, our age, our habits, our culture and a lot of other factors that make us unique.

In the equation of happiness, the body is a crucial factor, because we are always body, we feel pain, pleasure, tiredness, we like or dislike our bodies, we dress them with sizes and fashions, the body is the first thing we show just by the fact of walking into a room or shaking someone's hand. Although we are beings of ideas, of thoughts, the body is our way of entering the world, the first contact, the eyes of others look at faces and bodies, and we look at others: their presence, their bearing, their majesty, their shyness. When we wake up in the morning we look at our hands, our arms, we rub our eyelids and stretch our muscles. And when we brush ourselves in front of the mirror, there we are: skin, muscles, bones...

For many the obsession with the body becomes unhealthy, because they aspire to have a body that is not theirs. Our body is the one we have, we can not change it, although this sounds very elementary this is a truth that many obviate. This does not mean that we cannot adjust many things about our body, improve it (or make it worse if our habits are lousy), make it more agile, slimmer, rounder, stronger, but in the end it is the body we were born with. Not even the most invasive plastic surgery operations can take away our body (even if in many cases they deform it, it is still our body).

The well-being of the body is the well-being of the mind. The mind manifests itself through the body: when we talk, argue, walk, cry, laugh, breathe, digest or rest... our worries, desires and frustrations materialize through the channel of our body. Both are intimately linked, they are part of a delicate system; therefore, the wellbeing of one is the wellbeing of the other. We could spend ten pages defining what well-being is, but for the moment let's stick with the idea that everyone can reach a sincere definition through a deep inner examination (leaving aside stereotypes and social pressures) to know when one feels good, full, satisfied.

Let us not forget that well-being implies a process of acceptance. When we accept reality and enjoy it, we feel good and love life. Acceptance does not mean that we do not want to modify habits and even things we do not like to change things in our life and body (lose or gain some pounds, cut or paint our hair, become stronger or more flexible). Change is welcome as long as it is within the parameters of acceptance.

Accepting that our body is unique leads us to act to take care of it in the best possible way, regardless of its shape or size. In this process, we stop comparing ourselves to others. And when we feel good physically and mentally, everything in life seems easier. We feel more motivated, we have more energy and we feel happier and more satisfied. On the other hand, when our body and mind are out of balance, we feel tired, stressed and unmotivated.

Especially when you are younger, health seems a distant topic, but after a certain age, little details begin to appear, as in a car that has never been maintained. Health is synonymous with life, it is not a simple fashion. When we eat well, exercise and take care of our emotional state, we are reducing the risk of diseases and health problems in the future. In other words, we are taking care of our body, which is the container of our life.

This book is for all those people who want to feel good about themselves and find their own balance between body and mind. In the following pages we offer practical and realistic tools and advice on nutrition, exercise, rest and healthy habits.

Remember that the version of yourself is the one you decide to be. Fashions pass, but your body remains. Be intuitive and reasonable and you will see how you will achieve the physical and mental satisfaction that will make you have a fuller life.

WE ARE DUAL BEINGS

Our body and mind are a unit. Taking care of one means taking care of the other. When we exercise, we are not only strengthening our muscles and improving our cardiovascular health, but we are also releasing endorphins, the famous "happy hormones". These chemicals have the ability to reduce stress and anxiety, improve our mood and increase our overall sense of well-being. When we lack them, we feel down and discouraged, when we have them afloat we are full of energy and good vibes.

Exercise can also improve the quality of our sleep. By getting a good night's sleep, we wake up with more energy and vitality, which allows us to better face the challenges of everyday life. A good night's sleep helps regulate appetite and can improve our body's ability to process nutrients, which in turn has a positive impact on our physical health.

Emotional well-being is not limited to physical exercise. It also involves taking care of our mind and emotions. This can include practices such as meditation, yoga, therapy or simply taking the time to do activities that we enjoy and relax. Like exercise, these practices can reduce stress and anxiety, and improve our mental health. And emotional wellbeing has an impact on physical health, as many of the body's ailments are emotional in origin: stress, anger, boredom, hopelessness can cause illness if we do not control them.

It is crucial to pay attention to what we eat. A healthy, balanced diet can not only help us maintain a healthy weight and prevent disease, but it can also have an impact on our emotional well-being. Some nutrients, such as omega-3 fatty acids and tryptophan, have been associated with better mental health and a lower risk of depression.

Of course, taking care of our physical and emotional well-being is not always easy. We often find ourselves busy with our daily lives and don't seem to have time to exercise or cook healthy meals. In addition, it can be difficult to find the right balance between work, family and time for ourselves.

Taking care of ourselves is not a luxury, but a necessity. By dedicating time and attention to ourselves, we can improve our quality of life and be in better conditions to face the challenges that life presents us.

Why is it important to feel satisfied with our body?

When we feel satisfied with our body, we are more likely to take care of it and keep it in good shape. We take care of what we want. By being aware of this, then instead of seeing exercise and healthy eating as a punishment for our body, we are motivated to maintain a healthy lifestyle in the long run. In addition, feeling satisfied with our bodies can improve our self-esteem and confidence. When we feel good about ourselves, we are more likely to have a positive and confident attitude about life.

Feeling satisfied with our bodies can also help us overcome social and cultural pressure to have a "perfect" body. We live in a society that often bombards us with images and messages about what our bodies are supposed to look like. These ideals are often unattainable and even unhealthy for most people. There is a reason why they are ideals, because they belong to the world of ideas and not reality. Reality is what we can touch, the body that accompanies us day and night. By feeling satisfied with our own body, we can accept ourselves and our differences, and learn to appreciate beauty in all its forms.

Of course, feeling satisfied with our bodies is not easy for everyone. It can take time and effort to learn to accept ourselves and love our bodies as they are, but it is an important and necessary process for our physical and emotional health.

The mind-body connection

The mind and body are like a garden that we can either let wither or make bloom.

The body would be the soil of that garden. We need to feed it with the right nutrients, such as protein, vitamins and minerals, so that it can grow strong and healthy. Like a garden, we also need to exercise it to keep it in good shape. Exercise is like digging the soil of that garden, which allows the roots to grow deeper and the soil to oxygenate. It's like giving our body a good massage!

The mind and thoughts would be the plants in that garden. If we do not take proper care of them, they can wither. Like plants, we need to nourish our mind with positive ideas and activities, such as optimistic thoughts, relaxation, life projects and meditation. Otherwise, we can experience stress and anxiety, which are like weeds in our mental garden. So let's make sure we pull those weeds and let our mental flowers grow.

Just like in a garden, mind and body are connected, in fact we are dual beings. If our body is in good shape, our mind will be too. When we exercise, we release endorphins, which are like vitamins for our mental garden. They make us feel good and give us the energy to keep going. But if we don't take care of our mind, we can experience physical health problems. Anxiety and stress can increase the risk of heart disease, diabetes and other conditions. Let's make our mental garden one we love to visit and even show off to others.

If our body were a garden, exercise would be like the sun. Exercise is a way to keep our bodies moving and active. It helps us build muscle, strengthen bones and improve cardiovascular health. In addition, it can improve our mental and emotional health, reduce stress and anxiety, and make us feel good about ourselves. It's as if the sun is nourishing and feeding our body garden.

Food would be like rain in our body garden, which needs the right amount of water and nutrients to grow and flourish. Just as plants require water and nutrients to grow, our body needs healthy and nutritious foods to stay healthy. Healthy foods such as fruits, vegetables and lean proteins are rich in nutrients that our body needs to stay healthy. It is as if we are watering our body garden with water and fertilizer.

But if we eat processed and sugary foods, our bodies don't get the nutrients they need. Instead of feeling healthy and energized, we will feel tired, lethargic and cranky. Excessive consumption of these types of foods has been linked to an increased risk of chronic diseases such as obesity and diabetes. It is as if our body garden is receiving toxic industrial waste and is slowly drowning in it.

In summary, exercise and nutrition are two important factors in our physical and emotional health. Exercise helps us stay in good shape and improve our mental and emotional health. And food provides us with the nutrients our body needs to stay healthy and prevent disease. This way, we will have a beautiful and healthy body garden, so we can enjoy life to the fullest.

EMOTIONAL WELL-BEING

Emotional well-being is a vital part of our overall health, it is about feeling balanced, satisfied and able to face any challenge.

Have you ever felt emotionally drained, stressed or anxious? Well, emotional wellness is the exact opposite. It's when you feel happy, relaxed and calm. It also means that you can manage stress and anxiety effectively, and have healthy relationships with others. It also includes having purpose and meaning in our lives. It means having clear goals and objectives, and working to achieve them. When we have purpose, we find the motivation and satisfaction to keep going, even in the most difficult times. It is as if we were climbing a mountain, knowing that there is an incredible view at the top and that it is worthwhile to keep going despite the setbacks (which there will always be).

Emotional well-being is not something that is achieved overnight. It is an ongoing process that requires constant attention and effort. At times, we may feel overwhelmed or emotionally drained, but with practice and patience, we can develop the ability to manage our emotions effectively.

Thoughts and emotions influence our well-being. Sometimes, we underestimate the importance of what we think and feel, but they actually have a very big impact on our lives. Our thoughts are like seeds that we plant in our mind. If we plant negative thoughts, we will feel bad and not be in our best emotional state. But if we plant positive thoughts, like "I am capable" or "I am strong," then we will be in a better emotional state. It is as if we are planting a garden in our mind, and we have to plant the right seeds for beautiful flowers to grow.

Our emotions are like the weather in this mental garden. If we have negative thoughts, we may experience negative emotions such as sadness, anxiety or stress. On the other hand, if we plant positive thoughts, we can experience positive emotions such as happiness, joy and satisfaction. A garden needs a good climate to be at its best.

This is because our thoughts and emotions are connected. If we have negative thoughts, we experience negative emotions and vice versa. For example, if we have negative thoughts about ourselves, we may feel sad and worthless. But if we have positive thoughts, we may feel happy and confident. It is as if our thoughts are a light switch for our emotions.

But all is not lost if we have negative thoughts. We can change our thoughts and emotions through practice and effort, focus on the positive, practice gratitude and optimism, and thus train our mind to think more positively. It is as if we are teaching our mental garden to grow in a healthier and happier direction.

Strategies to manage stress and anxiety

Stress and anxiety can be a headache (literally). They're like a silent disease, but there are fun and effective strategies to manage them.

The first strategy is to do breathing exercises. Take a deep breath and exhale slowly. Repeat this process several times and you will feel your body begin to relax. You can also imagine that you are inhaling positive things, like the sun or the sea breeze, and exhaling negative things, like traffic or work. It's like doing yoga but without the mat.

Another strategy is to laugh. Laughter is the best medicine, and it can reduce stress and anxiety. Sometimes all it takes to laugh is watching a funny movie, watching a comedy show, reading a funny book, or spending time with funny friends.

You can also do relaxing activities, such as reading a book of poems, taking a warm bath, listening to soft music or meditating. Find something that makes you feel relaxed and fulfilled. You can even try taking a nap. It's like a home spa, but without the exorbitant costs.

Another strategy is to do something creative, such as drawing, painting, or crafting. Find something you enjoy doing and spend time on it. One example is to make a scrapbook or a gratitude journal. It's like having an adult playtime.

Finally, changing your perspective on things and focusing on the positive can make a big difference in managing stress and anxiety. So think of situations for which you are grateful, focus on what you can control and let go of what is beyond your reach. It's like having good sunglasses on a cloudy day.

Mindfulness techniques to improve attention and concentration

Mindfulness is a concept that refers to being totally in the present moment, without our head in the future or in the past, but with maximum attention and concentration on what we are seeing or doing. There are many techniques to reach this state.

The first is conscious listening. Choose a song you like, and listen to each note and lyric with full attention. Focus on the melody, the words and the sounds of the instruments. If your mind wanders, refocus on the song. Enjoy the melody, the tone of voice, the background instruments, even the silences.

Another technique is the rain meditation. Sit in a comfortable place and close your eyes. Imagine that you are listening to the rain falling, and pay attention to the sounds and discover the patterns that occur. You can even play a recording of a rainfall and listen to it. If your mind wanders, refocus on that sound, the smells and sensations it evokes.

You can also try the visualization technique. Choose an image you like, such as a beach or a garden, and close your eyes. Imagine you are in that place, and pay attention to the details. If your mind wanders, refocus on the image.

Another practice is yoga or mindful stretching. Choose some simple yoga postures or stretches, and do them with mindfulness. Pay attention to your breathing and how your body feels in each posture. Your mind will try to think of something else, some unfinished task or worry, but as soon as that train of thought begins, focus back on your breathing and the posture.

Finally, try the mindful tasting. Choose a food that you like, and eat it with mindfulness. Pay attention to the flavors, texture and aromas of each bite. Enjoy it as if that dish was the first thing you tasted after days of fasting.

There are many fun mindfulness techniques that can help you improve your attention and concentration. Whether it's mindful listening, meditating, visualizing, yoga or stretching, or mindful eating, there's something for everyone!

You can design many more to suit you. The goal is to do everything with maximum focus and live the present in detail, with the maximum possible concentration. It is undoubtedly one of the most fulfilling ways to be in life.

MAINTAINING LONG-TERM WELL-BEING

Sometimes we have a "problem-solving" mentality where we only focus on solving a specific issue in the present moment, but we don't think about how to maintain long-term wellness.

When we maintain wellness throughout our lives, we are taking care of our body and mind. This means we are making healthy choices and taking steps to prevent health problems, for example, exercising regularly, eating a healthy diet, getting enough sleep and managing stress. Not only does this improve our quality of life, but it can also help us prevent chronic health problems such as heart disease, diabetes and cancer.

When we feel good physically and mentally for long and continuous periods we have more energy and are more productive, we are better able to concentrate and perform our tasks effectively. This can help us in our careers, relationships and personal goals.

On the other hand, maintaining long-term wellness can help us save time, money and stress in the future. When we prevent health problems and take good care of ourselves, we can avoid costly doctor visits and expensive medications. We can also avoid the stress and worry of dealing with chronic health problems, as these types of illnesses are not only problematic because of the disease itself, but because of all that it entails (expenses, debt, family worries, etc.).

Healthy habits are a lifestyle, not a quick fix. We need to embrace the process and be patient with ourselves. We can't expect to change our habits overnight, but if we are persistent and keep working on our long-term goals, we will eventually start to see results.

Consistency is key. It is to take, even one step at a time, but not to stop walking.

We must make healthy habits an integral part of our lifestyle and stay committed for the long term. At the end of the day, maintaining healthy habits and mind-body balance is a journey and not a goal. We must enjoy the journey and celebrate our accomplishments along the way.

To achieve consistency, we need to make our healthy habits fun and engaging. Just like when we listen to music to make exercise more appealing, we need to find ways to make our healthy habits more exciting and engaging.

One way to do this is to find activities that we enjoy and like to do. If we hate working out at the gym, why not try something different like yoga or dancing? If we don't like eating boring salads, we can try adding different ingredients or trying new healthy recipes.

We can also make our healthy habits a social experience, i.e., find friends who share our wellness interests, exercise together, share common reading and activities, or go out for healthy meals. This keeps us motivated and allows us to have a fun and social experience.

Set realistic and achievable objectives

Many times, we set goals that are impossible to achieve, which leads us to feel frustrated and unmotivated. That is why it is important to follow guidelines that allow us to set goals that are really achievable.

First, it is important to have a clear idea of what we want to achieve. Do we want to feel more relaxed? Do we want to improve our physical condition? Do we want to sleep better at night? Whatever our goal is, it is important to have it clear in our minds, because that is how we prepare ourselves to reach that place.

Next, we need to set specific and measurable goals. For example, if we want to improve our physical condition, instead of setting a general goal such as "I want to be fit", we can set a more specific and measurable goal, such as "I want to be able to run 30 minutes without stopping in the next month". This way, we can measure our progress and see how far we have come.

It is also important to set realistic goals. We cannot expect to achieve significant change overnight, such as saying we want to run a marathon next weekend if we have not done any physical activity for years. Unrealistic goals end in frustration and abandonment to pursue other goals. Therefore, we must be realistic and set goals that are achievable within a given time frame. In this way, we can feel motivated and committed to work towards our goal.

Some realistic and achievable objectives may include:

- Exercise for 30 minutes at least 3 times a week.
- Add a serving of fruits and vegetables to each meal.
- Practice meditation for 5 minutes a day.
- Eat one less serving per day of processed foods and refined sugars.
- Practice gratitude by writing down three things you are grateful for each night before you go to sleep.
- Take a 20-minute walk during lunch.
- Take a relaxing bath before going to bed 2 times a week.
- Have one less alcoholic drink at a time.
- Make a weekly list of tasks and priorities to better manage stress.

Each person is unique, and your goals should be too. Find what works best for you and adjust your goals as needed. Keep a positive attitude and celebrate your accomplishments along the way.

In addition, it is important to be flexible and adjust our goals if necessary. Sometimes, unforeseen events or changes in our lives can come up that prevent us from achieving our goals. If one day we don't achieve what we set out to do, it doesn't mean that our plan has fallen apart, it's just a day or two where we've set aside our goals. We can always get back on track.

The role of motivation in long-term wellbeing.

Just as a seed needs solid soil to grow, we need a positive attitude and a belief in ourselves to cultivate our motivation. We must regularly remind ourselves that we are capable of achieving what we set out to do.

We also need to surround ourselves with supportive people, like the bees that pollinate our plants. Just as they help flowers to grow, surrounding ourselves with supportive people helps us to maintain our motivation in the long run.

We must find ways to keep ourselves interested and excited, such as changing our exercise routines or our food recipes from time to time, just like when we change our plants in the garden. If we do the same thing every day, we can get bored and lose motivation.

Gamifying our physical and mental wellness goals can be a fun and effective way to keep us motivated and engaged. Gamification involves adding game elements to our everyday tasks to make them more interesting and challenging. Here are some ways to gamify our physical and mental wellness goals:

Use wellness apps: There are many wellness apps that allow us to set goals, track our progress and earn points and rewards. These apps can be a fun way to gamify our goals and motivate us to achieve them.

Set challenges: Setting challenges for ourselves can be a fun way to gamify our goals. We can set challenges for ourselves, such as running a certain distance in a certain time or doing a certain amount of push-ups, reading a book every week, eating vegetables as many times a day...

Create a reward game: We can create a reward game for ourselves, where we earn points for every time we exercise or eat healthy food. After earning a certain amount of points, we can redeem them with something we want.

Find an exercise partner: Finding an exercise partner can be a fun way to gamify our fitness goals. We can set challenges between us, and the one who loses, for example, must pay for the other's lunch to help us with some household chore.

Use board games: There are many board games that focus on health and wellness, such as card games that teach us about nutrition or board games that motivate us to exercise. These games can be a fun way to gamify our physical and mental wellness goals.

To have a healthy and beautiful garden, we need to have a strong and constant motivation. To achieve this, we must have a positive attitude and believe in ourselves, surround ourselves with supportive people, and find new and exciting ways to keep ourselves interested.

DISCOVER YOUR BODY

Have you ever felt like you don't really know your own body or that you're not sure how to properly train or nourish it? Well, this is something that happens to many people.

Discovering your body involves knowing its structure, needs and limitations. When you know your body, you can design a training and nutrition program that is right for you and that will help you reach your goals effectively.

In addition, knowing your body helps you identify the areas you need to work on the most. If you know you have weaknesses in a certain body part, for example, you can design a training program that focuses on strengthening those specific areas or skills.

Another reason it is important to discover your body is that it allows you to prevent injury and illness. When you know your limitations and needs, you can avoid workouts or movements that can cause injury. You can also detect health problems early and seek medical attention if necessary.

Body types and body composition

The human body is an incredibly complex and diverse machine, and each individual has his or her own body type and body composition. Knowing these differences can be essential to achieving your fitness and health goals.

Broadly speaking, there are three body types: ectomorph, mesomorph and endomorph. In this part of the book, we will explore each body type and its specific characteristics, all in a friendly and easy to understand manner.

Ectomorph

If you are an ectomorph, you may have difficulty gaining muscle or weight, but that doesn't mean you can't have a strong, healthy body.

Characteristics of the ectomorph body:

- Thin and slender bone structure
- Elongated bones and muscles
- Rapid metabolism
- Low body fat
- Difficulty gaining weight and muscle mass

Ectomorphs tend to have good muscle definition and an athletic appearance, often with a flat, well-defined abdomen. They also have a fast metabolism, which means they can eat more without gaining weight. However, the difficulty in gaining weight and muscle mass can be frustrating for ectomorphs who want to develop their bodies. In addition, having low body fat can be a challenge for maintaining energy and health.

Ideal nutrition for an ectomorph body:

Consume enough calories: Since ectomorphs have a fast metabolism, they need to consume enough calories to maintain their weight. Try to consume calorie-rich foods such as nuts, avocados, lean meats and whole dairy.

Eat high quality protein: Protein is essential for building muscle mass. Try to consume enough high-quality protein such as eggs, lean meats, fish and legumes.

Consume complex carbohydrates: Carbohydrates are an important source of energy for the body. Try to consume complex carbohydrates such as brown rice, whole wheat pasta, whole wheat bread and vegetables.

Control portion sizes: It is important to control portion sizes to avoid excess calories and maintain a healthy body.

Ideal physical activity for an ectomorph body:

Weight training: Resistance exercises and weight lifting are essential for building muscle mass. Try to focus on compound exercises such as squats, bench presses, pull-ups and deadlifts. If you are a beginner you need an instructor to guide you on the correct technique and how to dose the loads to achieve sustained and lasting progress.

Get enough rest: It is important to allow muscles to rest and recover after a workout. Rest 48 to 72 hours before training the same muscles again. It is in recovery that broken muscle fibers regenerate, gradually increasing in size.

Don't overdo cardio: Although cardiovascular exercise is important for maintaining good cardiovascular health, ectomorphs should be careful

not to overdo cardio, as this can burn calories and prevent weight gain.
Listen to your body's signals: hunger, satiety, pain, etc. To each signal you must give the appropriate response: do not go hungry, do not go thirsty, rest to recover.

Mesomorph

If you are a mesomorph, you may have a muscular bone structure and a fast metabolism, which allows you to build muscle easily.

Characteristics of the mesomorphic body:

- Wide and muscular bone structure
- Shoulders and hips in proportion
- Rapid metabolism
- Increased muscle mass
- Low body fat

Mesomorphs have a muscular bone structure and a fast metabolism, which allows them to build muscle easily. In addition, they have a good muscle to body fat ratio, which gives them an athletic appearance. But, if they do not take care of their nutrition and physical activity, mesomorphs have a tendency to gain weight easily.

Ideal nutrition for a mesomorph body:

Eat enough protein: Protein is essential for maintaining and building muscle mass. Try to consume enough high-quality protein, such as eggs, lean meat, fish, legumes and low-fat dairy products.

Include complex carbohydrates: Carbohydrates are an important source of energy for the body. Include complex carbohydrates in your diet, such as brown rice, whole wheat pasta, whole wheat bread and vegetables.

Portion control: Although mesomorphs have a good muscle to body fat ratio, it is important to control portions to avoid excess calories and maintain a healthy body.

Ideal physical activity for a mesomorph body:

Strength training: Resistance exercises and weight lifting are essential for maintaining and building muscle mass. Try to focus on compound exercises. Incorporate cardio: Cardio is important for maintaining good cardiovascular health and burning calories. Incorporate activities such as running, swimming, biking or dance classes.

Vary your training: To avoid plateauing, it is important to vary your training every four to six weeks. This way your body will respond better to a new stimulus rather than the usual.

Endomorph

If you have an endomorph body, you may have a tendency to store body fat, especially in the abdominal area, and you may have a slower metabolism.

Characteristics of the endomorphic body:

- Tendency to store body fat, especially in the abdominal area
- Slower metabolism
- Large bones and joints
- Wide and rounded waist
- Short legs and arms compared to the torso

Endomorphs usually have good bone structure, which gives them a solid, robust appearance. They also have greater physical endurance than other body types. They also have a tendency to store body fat, especially in the abdominal area, and their metabolism tends to be slower.

Ideal nutrition for an endomorph body:

Control carbohydrate intake: Endomorphs tend to have a slower metabolism and store body fat easily, so it is important to control the intake of simple carbohydrates, such as sugar and white flour. Instead, consume complex carbohydrates, such as vegetables and fruits, brown rice, whole grain bread and legumes.
Eat enough protein: Protein is essential for maintaining and building muscle mass. Try to

consume enough high-quality protein, such as eggs, lean meat, fish, legumes and low-fat dairy products.

Include healthy fats: Healthy fats, such as olive oil, avocado, nuts and seeds, are important for health and weight loss.

Ideal physical activity for an endomorph body:

Strength training: Resistance exercises and weight lifting are essential for maintaining and building muscle mass, which helps increase metabolism and burn fat. Try to focus on compound exercises such as squats, bench presses, pull-ups, dips and deadlifts. Muscle gain creates a residual calorie-burning effect. That is, the more muscle you build, the more calories you will burn even at rest.
Prioritize cardio: Cardiovascular exercise is important for maintaining good heart health and burning calories. Incorporate activities such as walking, running, biking, dance classes or swimming. It is important that it is high-impact cardio, meaning it gets your heart rate up. This will burn more calories in less time.

Listen to your body's signals: hunger, satiety and pain

Often, we are so busy with our lives that we don't take the time to pay attention to our body's signals, which can lead to poor eating habits and physical injuries.

Listening to your hunger and satiety is important to maintain healthy eating and avoid overeating. If you are distracted by other things while eating, you may not realize when you are full and end up eating more than you need to. Therefore, it is important to pay attention to how your body feels while eating and stop when you feel satisfied.

Listening to the signs of pain is crucial to avoid physical injury. Often, we ignore pain and continue to exercise or do activities that can make the injury worse. It is important to stop when you feel pain and allow your body to recover before continuing with any activity.

In addition, listening to your body's signals can also help you become more connected to yourself. By paying attention to how you feel physically and emotionally, you can identify the factors that make you feel good and those that cause you stress or anxiety.

So how can you start listening to your body's signals? Here are some suggestions:

Pay attention to your body while eating: Savor each bite and stop when you feel satisfied.

Pause during exercise if you feel pain. Do not force yourself to continue if you feel pain, take a break and allow yourself to recover before continuing.

Take a pause in your day to review how you feel. Take a few minutes during the day to evaluate your physical and emotional state, to analyze if you are giving your best, check your enthusiasm and ask yourself if it is really the day you want to have, and know that if you can't change it you can think of medium-term measures to modify some things in your environment.

In summary, listening to your body's signals is important to maintain a healthy diet, avoid physical injuries and be more motivated and relaxed. Remember that your body is your temple and deserves to be cared for and listened to.

Acceptance and self-love: how to work on our relationship with our body

In another of our books (*Look At Yourself And Accept Who You Are*) we talked extensively about acceptance, its benefits and the steps to achieve it to the fullest. Here we will only recapitulate some basic principles regarding body wellness.

To accept yourself is to appreciate the person you are, with all your virtues and flaws. It is to feel more confident and comfortable with ourselves, instead of worrying about what others think. It is to have self-love as a product of self-worth and knowing that we are unique.

Sometimes, it can be difficult to accept and love ourselves, but it is important to remember that we are all different and that is what makes us special. There will always be people who criticize or judge us, but the most important thing is that we learn to love and accept ourselves as we are.

Many compare themselves to others as a way to validate their physical appearance. As we saw, body types are different and within those three ranges there are endless variations. While you can bring out your greatest potential within your typology, the truth is that you can't change it to look like someone else if your build is different. It is true that in most cases you can lose weight or gain weight, increase your muscle, become stronger or more flexible. But if you are looking to look like a specific model you will most likely get frustrated and feel bad about yourself.

Perfection is as subjective as the goals you set for yourself, and should not be an imposition of the fads of the moment. That's what body acceptance is all about, knowing that you can make many adjustments that make you feel better, but also accepting that there are things that cannot change unless you subject yourself to physical and mental stress with potentially dire consequences (extreme weight loss, absurd training challenges, high-risk cosmetic surgery).

If you love yourself as you are and are aware of how you can realistically be, you will naturally look for ways to eat better, exercise more regularly and do activities that you enjoy. If you start from a deep-seated nonconformity, it will be more difficult to take care of your body. Remember that we take care of what we love and neglect what we despise.

Therefore, working on our relationship with our body is essential for our physical and emotional well-being. Some practices that can help you find that path of balance are:

Practice gratitude: Being grateful for the good things we have in our life and in our body is an excellent way to improve our relationship with our body. Being grateful for our health, for our well-functioning organs and for every part of our body helps us to value and respect it.

Paying attention to ourselves: Learning to listen to our body's signals, such as hunger, thirst, tiredness, helps us to take proper care of it. When we pay attention to our body's needs and attend to them, we create a healthier and more respectful relationship. Knowing which foods do not agree with us, which sleep and exercise schedules are uncomfortable, and at what times of the day cravings are confused with hunger will help us to modify patterns in a conscious and intelligent way.

Move: Our body is a machine designed to move. Exercise is not an additional and dispensable activity, but we should try to move as much as we can: walking, climbing stairs, getting up, bending down are verbs that we should execute as many times as we can. Eight-hour-a-day office jobs go against this principle; and besides causing health problems and stress, they train the body to be passive when it evolved for constant movement. If you make it conscious that you should move, you will look for the occasion to do it more often: avoid the elevator to just go up a few floors, avoid ordering lunch at home if you can walk a few blocks, enjoy a walk aimlessly just for the pleasure of moving your legs. Ideally, you should also introduce some training exercise sessions: weights or some sport. You will see that a body in motion always asks for more movement.

Respecting ourselves: Treating our body with affection and respect is fundamental to improve our relationship with it. Talking to ourselves in a kind and positive way, taking care of our skin and hair, admiring a particular detail about ourselves, dressing in comfortable clothes that make us feel good, are small actions that can help us cultivate a more loving relationship with our body.

Working on our relationship with our body requires daily practices that help us to accept and love it as it is. Sometimes this love is learned in childhood, sometimes we have to reinforce it with daily practices until this respect and affection for us becomes so natural that we will do everything possible to be well.

HEALTHY NUTRITION

Healthy nutrition is nutrition that includes a variety of fresh, natural foods that provide a good amount of essential nutrients to the body. This is achieved through a combination of foods rich in protein, complex carbohydrates, healthy fats, fiber, vitamins and minerals; as well as keeping processed foods rich in trans fats and sugars at bay. Healthy nutrition also involves eating in adequate and balanced portions and maintaining adequate hydration.

It's not about obsessing over a perfect diet but being reasonably flexible. Allowing yourself to indulge occasionally and enjoying a cheat meal now and then, without guilt or regret, is part of healthy but realistic eating.

A balanced and varied diet provides us with the essential nutrients we need to keep our bodies healthy and functioning well. These nutrients include proteins, carbohydrates, fats, vitamins and minerals. Each of them has an important function in our body, from repairing tissues to maintaining our immune system. Eating well in healthy terms can help us prevent chronic diseases such as diabetes, cardiovascular conditions, high blood pressure and even some types of cancer.

A balanced and varied diet does not mean that we should deprive ourselves of the foods we like. In fact, including some not-so-healthy foods in our diet from time to time is perfectly normal and can be part of a healthy lifestyle. The key is to find balance and moderation.

Some recommendations to achieve a balanced and varied diet include:

- Consume a variety of fresh, whole foods such as fruits, vegetables, lean proteins and whole grains.
- Limit consumption of processed foods high in sugar, saturated fat and sodium. The less packaged products you consume the better.
- Moderate the consumption of alcohol and sugary beverages such as soft drinks or unnatural juices.
- Plan meals in advance and carry healthy snacks to avoid being tempted to eat less healthy foods. Sometimes, with the excuse of a hurry, the easiest thing to do is to eat a snack, since this is what is in abundance in convenience stores.

Foods that make us feel good

Some foods are called "comfort foods" or "happy foods," but why do they make us feel that way?

First of all, it is important to clarify that the foods that make us feel good are not necessarily the least healthy foods. In fact, many of them are rich in nutrients and can be part of a balanced and healthy diet. What makes them special is their ability to activate certain areas of the brain that produce a feeling of satisfaction.

One of the main foods that make us feel good are complex carbohydrates, such as whole grains, fruits and vegetables. These foods contain sugars and fiber that are slowly released into the bloodstream, providing us with long-lasting, stable energy. In addition, complex carbohydrates also stimulate the production of serotonin, a neurotransmitter that makes us feel relaxed and happy.

Another group of foods in this category are those containing healthy fats, such as olive oil, avocados, nuts and fatty fish such as tuna and salmon. These foods are rich in omega-3 fatty acids, which have been shown to have positive effects on mental health and can reduce inflammation in the brain.

Some foods contain tryptophan, an amino acid that is converted to serotonin in the brain. These foods include turkey, chicken, eggs, cheese, tofu and nuts. Therefore, consuming these foods can help us increase serotonin levels in the brain and improve our mood.

On the other hand, there are foods that give us a short-lived but addictive feeling of euphoria. A candy bar, a sugary soda and industrial pastries in general produce a momentary happiness that soon evaporates and leaves us wanting more. That is why we should avoid them and look for those healthy foods that fill us with lasting energy and good mood. Finding and incorporating these foods into your daily diet will make you feel satisfied and happy to be giving your beloved body good fuel.

Strategies for maintaining a healthy diet on a day-to-day basis

Sometimes it can be difficult to eat well in the midst of our busy lives and the overabundance of "cheap" junk food. We say "cheap" in quotation marks because, although the cost may be lower, in the long run it ends up being more expensive to eat a diet of this style because the expense in medical bills will come sooner or later if this is our predominant source of food.

It is important to plan your meals and prepare them ahead of time. You can cook several dishes at the same time so that you have enough healthy meals refrigerated for the entire week. Also, having meals already prepared will make it easier to make healthy choices when you are busy or tired.

Find recipes that are fun and exciting for you. Look for new ingredients that you haven't tried before or experiment with different ways of cooking your favorite foods. Change can be fun and will help you discover new foods and flavors.

Another strategy is to make food attractive. Try presenting your dishes in a suggestive and appetizing way, using plates and utensils with bright colors or adding some spices or herbs to give flavor and color to your dishes. Try to chop and distribute the vegetables in a way that brightens up the dish. A colorful dish is more eye-catching and its pleasure enters through the eyes.

It is important to buy healthy foods that you really like. The range of healthy foods is very varied and the truth is that we don't have to like them all. There are people who do not tolerate the smell or taste of cauliflower, eggplant, radishes, for example. It is not an obligation to consume them because there are many alternatives. The vegetable kingdom is much more varied than the animal kingdom when it comes to food. If you buy healthy foods that you do not like, it is likely that you will not eat them and end up opting for less healthy options, or that you will strengthen the prejudice that eating healthy is not pleasant.

And do not neglect hydration. At this point, the simplest and healthiest thing to drink is water. Natural juices are better than processed ones, but their excess represents a large intake of sugar, so their consumption should be moderate. Tea and coffee do not agree with everyone. So to keep our body hydrated and healthy, plain water is best. If you find it hard to drink enough water during the day you can add chia, lemon, basil leaves, cucumber, etc., for various flavors. In addition to its benefits, water can also be an effective way to reduce appetite and avoid overeating.

DIET MYTHS

Misinformation and myths can confuse people and lead them to make the wrong choices in many aspects of life, and food is no exception. This can lead to long-term health problems, such as nutritional deficiencies, digestion problems, hormonal imbalances, weight gain and chronic diseases.

In the information age, misinformation is rampant, so everything we read or hear has to be taken with a grain of salt, no matter how many times it has been repeated or if there are some supposed specialists who endorse such information.

For more than fifty years we have been hearing about the periodic appearance of the ultimate miracle diet. Each one replaces and contradicts the previous one. Some are fads for a few months and others fads that come and go every few years. It would not be surprising if at some point the diet of eating only seeds, only ostrich eggs or only mud becomes fashionable (perhaps there are already equally irrational proposals).

The truth is that a perfect diet, with immediate and sustained results that works for all bodies and cultures does not exist. There are dietary programs that have better results in certain body types, but around all that there are usually life habits, cultural context, genetics and many other factors.

Of course, there are accurate and healthy recommendations from nutrition experts; but these recommendations are usually personalized and above all balanced. A nutritionist who tells you that you should only eat zebu meat or oat flakes all your life (supported by some almost mythical explanation) is certainly not a good professional.

The dangers of restrictive and fad diets

Fad diets are usually the restrictive ones, because their extremism tends to captivate many more people as they are presented as something supposedly new and radical. Often, these diets promise quick results, but in reality they can be very dangerous for our physical and mental health, as they can create conflicts, frustration, manias and even depression.

There is no shame in ever falling into the trap of following a miracle diet or consuming magic shakes. It is really difficult not to succumb to the power of marketing. It is natural to want results in a short time at the cost of supposed sacrifices.

The truth is that restrictive diets are not sustainable in the long term. And the idea of a diet is that it should be a habit, something that comes naturally to us. And what is natural is what each culture has as its point of balance, where there is no room for unbridled excess (as in our time of overabundance of addictive junk food) or voluntary deprivation.

So how to eat healthy? The answer lies in balance. Ancient cultures (or those on the fringes of contemporary society) ate what was available, what they could hunt and fish, what they could gather. They didn't voluntarily choke or starve themselves. They didn't have mid-afternoon cravings that they quickly solved with a packed lunch. They ate just enough, what their bodies needed.

Today's society has perverted the concept of nutrition by making us repudiate the body we have and making us wish we had the body of a distant ideal. On the one hand, there is a lot of junk food available and relatively cheap; and on the other hand, magic pills and extreme and miraculous diets that want to combat these disorders with dangerous and unrealistic promises. The food and health machinery is a snake that bites its own tail, a detrimental cycle that we must make an effort to get out of.

By limiting the amount of food we eat, we also limit the essential nutrients our bodies need to function properly. This can lead to nutritional deficiencies and affect our long-term health. And not all bodies function well by only eating meat and seeds, or only eating fruits and raw foods.

In addition, some fad diets often force us to eliminate entire food groups, such as carbohydrates or fats. This can lead to an unhealthy obsession with food and a negative relationship with eating. Another danger of restrictive diets is that they are often temporary and are not sustainable in the long term. Once we stop following the diet, it is easy to return to our old eating habits and regain the lost weight and actually gain excess weight.

Dietary restriction can lead to obsessive thoughts about food and guilt about eating certain foods. In addition, fad diets often promote an unrealistic body image and can affect our self-esteem and self-confidence.

Food should be a pleasure, a festive act, not a sin or an act that makes us feel bad.

Common myths about eating and weight loss

One of the most common myths is that in order to lose weight, we must follow an extremely low-calorie diet. While it may seem logical that by drastically reducing our caloric intake we will lose weight faster, this is not necessarily true. In fact, a very low-calorie diet can actually slow down our metabolism and make it more difficult to lose weight in the long run. For the body seeks balance and learns to conserve its fat reserves during this induced austerity. And in fact, when we increase calories again, they add up to much more than they did previously.

Another common myth is that we should avoid certain food groups to lose weight, such as carbohydrates or natural fats. In reality, all food groups are important and necessary for a healthy, balanced diet. Eliminating food groups can lead to nutritional deficiencies and affect our long-term health.

It is also often said that in order to lose weight we must exercise intensely and strenuously every day. While exercise is important for physical and mental health, it is important to find a balance and exercise in a way that is sustainable and healthy for our bodies. Over-exercising can lead to injury and burnout, which can affect our ability to stick to a long-term exercise plan. Unless we are elite athletes with an upcoming competition, our exercise plan should be demanding but not earth-shattering.

When it comes to seeking a balanced and sustainable diet, it is important to take a holistic approach that includes a variety of healthy and nutritious foods. Among them are:

Focus on whole foods: Instead of processed and packaged foods, try to focus on whole, fresh foods. This includes fruits, vegetables, whole grains, lean proteins and healthy fats. Think about everything your ancestors ate over a hundred years ago, or a thousand years ago: there weren't packaged foods of all sizes, flavors and colors waiting for them around every corner. They ate real food.

Balance your macros: A balanced and sustainable diet should include a good combination of macronutrients, i.e. proteins, carbohydrates and healthy fats. This helps to maintain stable blood sugar levels and keep us satiated for longer.

Try different foods and recipes: To avoid getting bored of the same foods, try different options and recipes. You can search online or in cookbooks to find healthy and delicious ideas to help you vary your diet. In today's overabundance, there are people who share good knowledge, varied and quality recipes. Don't just take the opinion of a couple of *influencers*, there is much more. By having a wide range of varied information, you will learn to distinguish quackery from common sense.

Eat mindfully: Learn to pay attention to your body's signals of hunger and satiety. Eat slowly, enjoying each bite and making sure you feel satisfied without feeling too full. It's a bit like what we discussed a few pages back about *mindfulness*, but applied to the act of eating.

Organize your meals in advance: If you prepare some dishes in advance or delegate someone else to do it, you will always have something healthy and appetizing in your refrigerator. There are many services of people dedicated to prepare customized menus per week. It is a much better investment than eating on the street, where sometimes time and circumstances do not leave us many options to choose from.

In short, balanced and sustainable eating is about taking a holistic approach that includes a variety of healthy and nutritious foods. By focusing on whole foods, balancing your macros, trying different options and recipes, eating mindfully and organizing your meals in advance, you can ensure that your eating is sustainable in the long term and helps you reach your health and body-loving goals.

EXERCISE FOR WELLNESS

Exercise is not only beneficial to our physical health, but it can also have a great impact on our emotional well-being. When we exercise, our brain releases endorphins, which are hormones that make us feel good, happy and relaxed. In addition, regular exercise can reduce stress and anxiety levels, improve sleep quality, increase self-esteem and self-confidence, and improve our ability to concentrate and remember.

Exercise can help us reduce stress and anxiety. Have you ever felt that feeling of release and euphoria after a strenuous workout? We already made reference to endorphins or the so-called "happiness hormones". Although it sounds paradoxical, they are a stimulus that energizes and relaxes us at the same time, and by the way we want more of it every time we experience them. Indeed, finding the physical activity that you like the most, and if possible in the company of like-minded people, can become one of those good addictions. Yes, there are good addictions, and exercise is one of them.

In addition, exercise can also improve the quality of our sleep by increasing the amount of time we spend in deep sleep, which helps us feel more rested and refreshed when we wake up. Tiring our body is an effective tool to then rest better. Today's society focuses on tiring and entertaining only our mind, hence the abundance of sleep problems today.

Exercise can help us reduce the risk of heart disease, diabetes and obesity, among other health conditions. Even if there is a genetic predisposition to some of these diseases, constant physical activity is an important factor in moderating the impact of these predispositions. It is not a magic formula, but it plays in our favor.

By exercising regularly, we can also improve our cardiovascular and muscular endurance, allowing us to perform daily activities with greater ease, as well as avoid injuries as we age. Old age is inevitable, but not active old age with a body capable of performing most daily and recreational activities.

We have already mentioned that our body is a movement machine. It is true that with age certain activities may become more limited, but this does not mean that our destiny is to be prostrate. Training when you are young is a guarantee of mobility (and therefore independence and well-being) for your future self.

On the other hand, it is never too late to start. It is not a question of someone in his seventies becoming an Olympic gymnast overnight; but it is feasible and real that in a relatively short time, someone in his third or fourth age can undertake training appropriate to his abilities and progress in it.

There are a multitude of exercises and each one can benefit our health in a different way. So it's relatively simple to create a workout plan tailored to your personal needs and tastes, making it easy to incorporate it into your daily routine and maintain it over the long term. Whether you prefer yoga, running, weight lifting or any other type of physical activity, this chapter will help you understand the wellness benefits of exercise and how you can make it part of your lifestyle.

Types of exercise: cardio, strength, flexibility

There are three main types of exercise we can do to improve our health and well-being: cardiovascular, strength and flexibility exercise. Each has unique benefits and can help us achieve different goals.

Cardiovascular exercise, or **cardio** as it is commonly called, is any type of exercise that increases our heart rate and makes us breathe faster. Some common examples of cardio are running, swimming, cycling and dancing.

This type of activity improves our cardiovascular health by strengthening our heart and lungs. It can also help us burn calories and lose weight.

Cardio can also have benefits for our emotional well-being. When doing cardio, our body releases endorphins, which make us feel good and help us reduce stress and anxiety.

Doing cardio often gives a feeling of freedom, energy and revitalization. There is something about running outdoors or dancing in a class that simply brings a feeling of happiness.

We are movement machines and also running machines. The design of our muscles, tendons, bones is made to eventually, several times in life, have to make a fast run. We evolved by running to save our lives or running to hunt for our food. That must be why cardiovascular exercise connects us to that essential part of our nature.

Strength exercises involve working our muscles against some resistance (either the force of gravity or our own weight or that of barbells and discs), for example, lifting weights or doing push-ups.

Strength training is not just for Olympic competitors, bodybuilders or construction workers. To a greater or lesser extent we all require a certain amount of strength for everyday activities.

These exercises strengthen our muscles and bones, which is especially important as we age and lose muscle mass and bone density. They also help us improve our posture and prevent injuries to our back and other muscles and joints.

Strength training can also have benefits for our mental and emotional health. As we realize our strength and physical progress, we can improve our self-esteem and self-confidence. That feeling of moving, pushing or lifting something heavy conveys a sense of power that also benefits us emotionally.

Strength is not something exclusive to men. Women also have and need strength.

To work on flexibility we must stretch and move our muscles and joints through a full range of motion. This helps us to improve our mobility, prevent injuries, rectify our posture and relieve muscle and joint pain.

Additionally, flexibility exercise can have benefits for our mental and emotional health. By doing stretching and mobility exercises, we can reduce stress and anxiety and improve our relaxation and concentration.

Having flexibility will make you feel more limber and in tune with your body. Plus, stretching and mobility exercises are a great way to relax after an intense strength or cardio workout.

How to design a training plan tailored to your needs and tastes

A workout plan should be challenging, but you should also like it, like everything in life. Fortunately, there is a wide variety of physical activities to do individually, in pairs or in groups.

There are specialists who can help you design training plans, with the right guidance to help you stay injury-free, progress and have fun.

Following these tips you can have the ideal scenario to make yours. Of course, if you need something very specific, have a special condition, or are in rehabilitation, a specialist will be the best person to guide you.

Make a plan that you can stick to for the long term, not just for a few weeks. This way, you can create a healthy lifestyle and maintain your results over the long term.

Vary your workouts. Variety is key to avoid boredom and maintain motivation. Try different types of activities, such as strength training, yoga, pilates, running, among others. In addition, varying your workouts will help you work different muscle groups and prevent injuries.

Don't forget to warm up and stretch. Warming up and stretching are essential to prevent injuries and improve flexibility. Spend a few minutes before and after each session to perform these exercises.

Listen to your body. Sometimes our body tells us that we need a rest day or that we need to reduce the intensity of our training. Learn to listen to your body and make the necessary adjustments to your training plan. If you are honest you will know when you need and can give more, and when you should take a break or change activity.

Setting realistic goals will help you stay motivated and avoid frustration. Instead of setting a goal to lose 10 pounds in a month, set a goal to lose half a pound per week. It will take longer, but it will come.

Find a training partner. This can be very motivating because you will share your accomplishments and support each other during difficult times.

Remember that every body is different and what works for one person may not work for another. Find what works for you and enjoy the process of reaching your goals. The rewards of running one more mile, lifting one more pound, kicking a ball harder than before are the best rewards for someone who trains. It's a challenge against yourself.

THE IMPORTANCE OF BUILDING MUSCLE

Have you ever wondered why some people can eat a lot without gaining weight while others gain weight easily? The answer lies in metabolism and muscle building.

Metabolism is the process by which our body converts food into energy. If you have a fast metabolism, your body burns calories faster and it is easier to lose weight. On the other hand, if you have a slow metabolism, your body burns calories more slowly and it is more difficult to lose weight.

But how can we speed up our metabolism? This is where building muscle mass comes into play. Muscle is more metabolically active than fat, which means that the more muscle we have, the more calories we burn at rest. In other words, our body will continue to burn calories even when we are sitting on the couch watching a movie or reading a book.

Strength training for muscle building not only helps us speed up our metabolism, but also helps us maintain strong bones and prevent injuries. So, if you want to increase your metabolism and improve your body composition, you should include strength training in your exercise routine. Your muscles will thank you for it.

In addition, muscles can also help us fight fatigue and increase our capacity to perform daily activities, making us more active.

Now, while many men are frustrated by how slow their muscle gain progress is, some women have an irrational fear of gaining too much muscle. The truth is that, depending on body type, muscle gain is usually not easy (it's usually easy to gain pounds in fat, but not in muscle).

But many women (although that perspective seems to be changing) shy away from weight training for fear of becoming a ball of muscle. Building muscle requires good training, a good diet and a lot of patience. Bulking up is not only a process that takes time, but also depends on body type. In general, if we train with weights and eat enough quality food, with an emphasis on protein and unprocessed carbohydrates, we will gain muscle progressively, but always within the patterns of our genetics.

Building muscle is not only healthy, but it gives every body (within its specific characteristics) a more toned and defined shape. Within a standard workout no one becomes a bodybuilder just by doing weights regularly.

We all have muscles, otherwise we would not be able to walk or scratch our bellies. Muscles are synonymous with health because they are reservoirs of energy and nutrients, they increase metabolism, reduce the risk of diseases such as diabetes, improve posture, prevent injuries... in short, they prolong life. Over the years, especially after 40-50 years of age, the body begins to lose muscle and keeping it becomes very difficult. That is why it is necessary to start building muscle as soon as possible.

Aesthetically, having muscle will make your clothes fit better, make you feel more energetic... make you feel more alive.

Myths about weight training and muscle development

"Women shouldn't lift heavy weights because they will get too muscular." The truth is that women don't have enough testosterone to build massive muscles like men. Lifting heavy weights will only make them stronger, more defined and toned.

"You should only train the muscles you see in the mirror." Wrong! The body is interconnected, and all muscles work together. It is important to train the whole body to maintain muscle balance and prevent injury. It's not just biceps and pecs, our muscular system is a complete system.

"You must do a lot of reps with little weight to tone muscles." Toning is just a fancy word to describe building muscle and losing fat. To achieve this, you need to lift heavy weights and do a moderate number of reps that will break down your muscle fibers and cause the muscle to grow. As we said, it's a slow process and you need to be patient.

"If you stop weight training, your muscles will turn to fat." This is biologically impossible. Muscle and fat are two different tissues that cannot transform into each other. If you stop weight training, your muscles will simply atrophy and become smaller.

"Weight training is dangerous and can cause injury". The truth is that we could injure ourselves in the shower or just going to buy bread. If weight training is done properly the risks of injury are minimal. It is important to learn the correct technique and start with weights appropriate to our level of experience and ability. In fact, lifting weights makes us less prone to injury in day-to-day activities.

But if you definitely do not like weights there are many options to gain muscle, such as calisthenics or practicing a sport like soccer, skating or swimming. Practiced in a sustained manner and with the proper advice will make us gain muscle.

Designing an effective weight training routine

Some of the most popular barbell exercises include squats, leg presses, deadlifts, shoulder presses, bicep curls and tricep extensions. Whether you're a beginner or advanced, there's always a weights routine to suit your needs. The purpose of this section is not to replace a professional trainer, but to familiarize you with the basic terms and techniques before joining a gym.

Always remember to warm up before any exercise and maintain proper technique to avoid injury.

Barbell Squats: Barbell squats are an incredible exercise for working your leg and gluteal muscles. To do them, start by holding a barbell with both hands or a barbell with discs on the trapezius of your back, with your feet shoulder-width apart. Slowly lower yourself down as if you were sitting in an imaginary chair, keeping your back straight and the weight on your heels. Then, return to the starting position and repeat the movement.

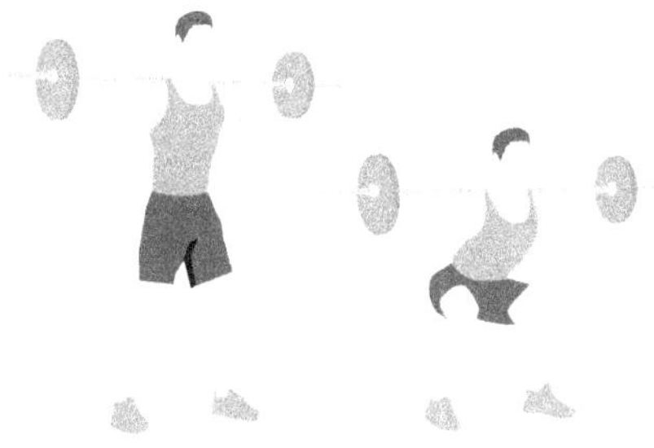

Leg press: Also known as leg press is another excellent exercise to strengthen the muscles of the legs and buttocks. If you don't have access to a leg press at the gym, you can do a weighted version at home. To do it, lie on your back with your knees bent and feet flat on the floor. Hold a dumbbell in each hand and lift your hips toward the ceiling, keeping your back straight and your abs contracted. Then, slowly lower yourself back down to the starting position and repeat the movement.

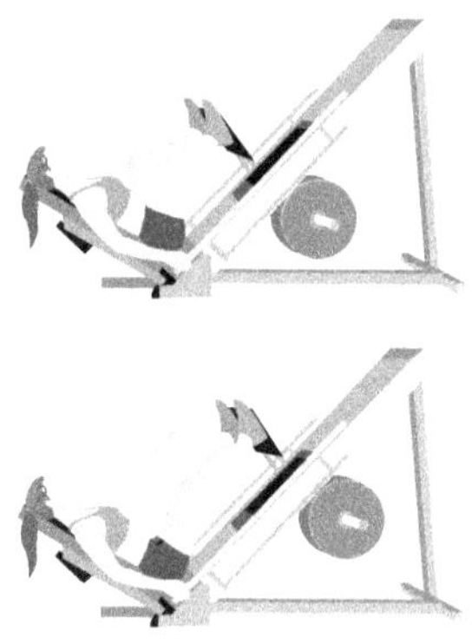

Deadlift: The deadlift is an excellent exercise for working your back and leg muscles. To do it, hold a dumbbell with both hands and place it in front of your thighs. Place your feet hip-width apart and slowly lower the weight to the floor, keeping your back straight and your abs contracted. Then return to the starting position.

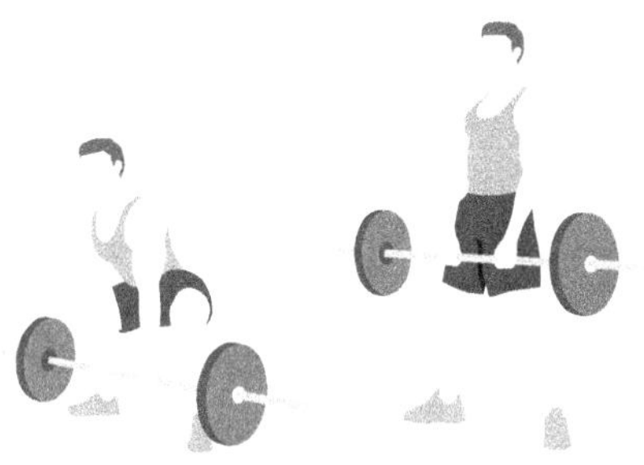

Shoulder press: The shoulder press is an excellent exercise for strengthening shoulder and arm muscles. To do it, hold a dumbbell in each hand and lift them to shoulder height, palms facing forward. Then, push the weights upward, fully extending your arms. Then, slowly lower the weights back to the starting position.

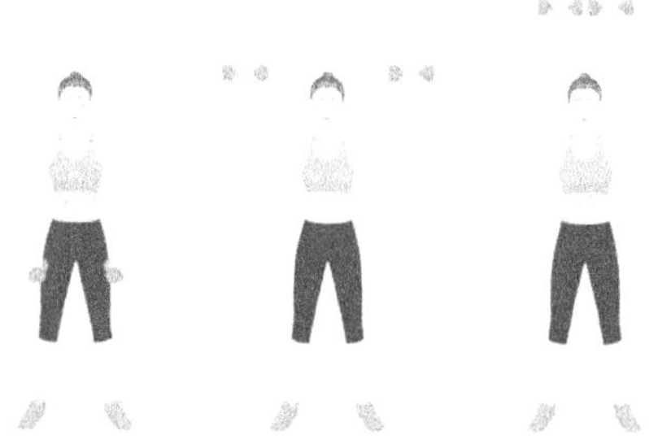

Biceps curl: The biceps curl is a classic exercise to work the arm muscles. To do it, hold a dumbbell in each hand and place them at the sides of your body, palms facing forward. Then, slowly lift the weights toward your shoulders, bending your elbows. Hold the position for a second and then lower the weights back to the starting position.

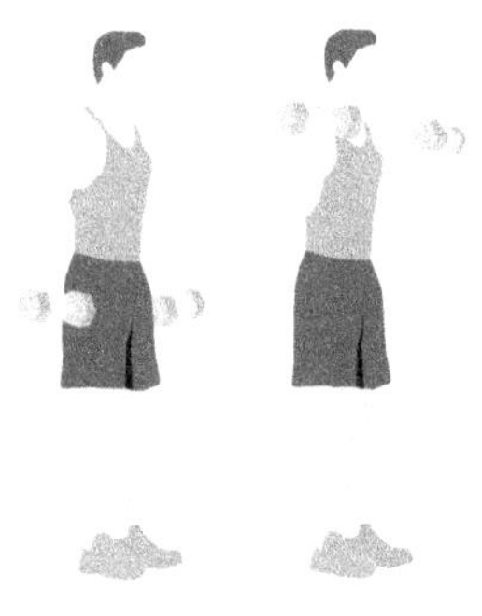

Triceps extensions: Triceps extensions are an excellent exercise to strengthen the muscles in the back of your arms. To do them, hold a dumbbell with both hands behind your head, with your elbows bent. Then, extend your arms upward, keeping your elbows close to your ears. Hold the position for a second and then lower the weights back to the starting position.

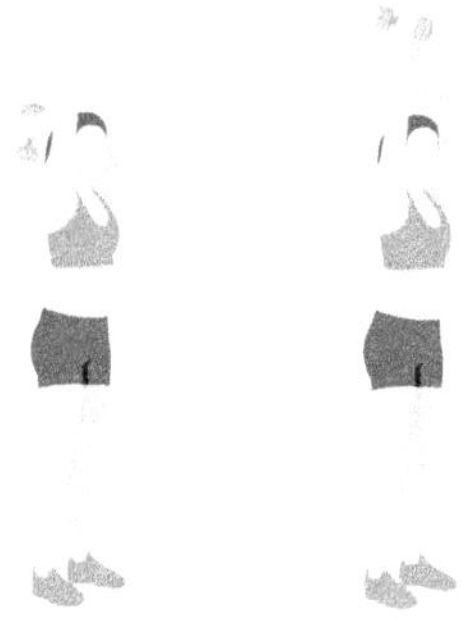

Protein, a key ally for muscle gain

Protein (whether of animal or vegetable origin) is the nutrient responsible for building and repairing muscle tissue. When we exercise, our muscles experience micro damage to their fibers that needs to be repaired. Protein helps repair this damage and build new muscle, resulting in increased muscle size and strength.

In addition, protein is essential to maintain a balanced and healthy diet. It helps control appetite, promotes satiety and stabilizes blood sugar levels. It can also help reduce the loss of muscle mass during a weight loss diet.

It is not necessary to consume large amounts of protein to gain muscle. The truth is the body can only synthesize a limited amount of protein at a time, so it is important to spread protein intake throughout the day. The standard is 0.4 to 0.6 grams of protein per pound of body weight throughout the day.

The amount of protein we need varies from person to person, depending on factors such as age, gender and level of physical activity. However, the important thing is to make sure we consume enough protein in our diet to meet our body's needs.

Animal protein is a common source of protein. Foods such as meat, poultry, fish and eggs are rich in animal protein. These foods contain essential amino acids, which our body cannot produce on its own and therefore must come from our diet.

On the other hand, there are also vegetable protein sources, such as legumes, nuts, seeds and some vegetables. While these protein sources do not contain all the essential amino acids, they can be combined to create a complete protein.

Protein supplements are a convenient and effective way to increase dietary protein intake, and one of the most popular is whey, also known as whey.

Whey is a complete protein, which means that it contains all the essential amino acids the body needs to build and repair muscle tissue. In addition, it is digested and absorbed quickly compared to other protein sources, making it an excellent choice for post-workout consumption when the body needs nutrients quickly to begin the recovery process.

It should be seen as a supplement to be used only in cases where, despite eating enough, we are not able to meet the daily dose of protein to gain muscle. In no case does whey replace real food.

HOME FITNESS TRAINING

There are circumstances that prevent us from exercising outdoors or joining a gym or sports center. In these contexts, exercising at home is a valid option that suits many people very well.

Working out at home can be just as effective and fun as working out in a gym. Faced with the excuse of lack of time and money, exercising in the comfort of your home is an excellent option for many. Plus, it gives you the freedom to choose the schedule that works best for you. You can exercise early in the morning, after work or even in the middle of the afternoon.

Another great advantage is that you can customize your training space. You can choose the music that motivates you the most or have the lighting that you like the most.

You don't need expensive equipment to do it. And in many cases you don't even need anything more than your own body. In general, with a simple mat, yoga mat or mat, and a pair of dumbbells you can do a wide variety of strength exercises, while cardio exercises such as jumping rope, burpees or jumping jacks do not require special equipment.

Of course, training at home can also have its disadvantages. For example, it can be difficult to maintain the motivation and discipline necessary to follow a consistent training plan. In addition, there may be distractions at home that prevent us from focusing on our training, such as the TV, food, phone calls, a visitor, or even the tempting comfort of our couch.

Another challenge with working out at home is the lack of adequate space. Some people may be fortunate enough to have a full gym in their home, but for most, space can be a constraint.

It must also be recognized that training at home can also be boring for some people. Unlike a gym, there is no community atmosphere or variety of activities and equipment available to keep our attention and motivation.

However, there are many options to overcome these disadvantages. For example, you can join online training groups through digital platforms, which will allow you to have the motivation and support of others.

You can also set up a regular workout schedule and try to eliminate distractions while exercising (if you can watch a movie while working out, you're either not paying attention to the movie or you're not working out well). And if you don't have access to weights, you can use your own body weight or buy some elastic bands which represent a fairly minor expense.

Although there is nothing like having a trainer or watching videos on the internet to better understand the mechanics of the exercises, we don't want to miss the opportunity to present you with some simple examples of exercises that you can do at home without using any equipment or material:

Squats: Stand with your feet shoulder width apart, lower your body as if you were going to sit on a chair and come back up.

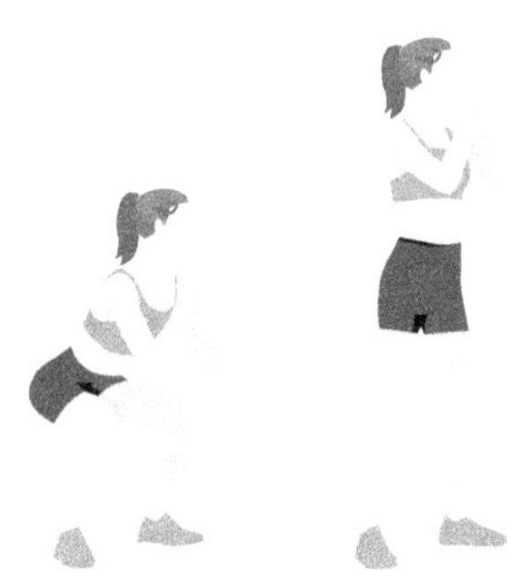

Stride: Take a big step forward with one leg, keep your knee bent and lower your hip until your back knee almost touches the ground. Step back up and repeat with the other leg.

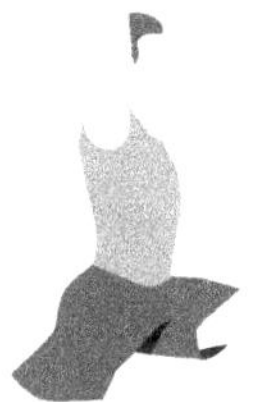

Plank: Lean on your forearms and toes, keep your body in a straight line and hold the position for a few seconds.

Push-ups: Get into a plank position with your hands under your shoulders, lower your body keeping your elbows close to your torso and come back up. If you can't do full push-ups, you can rest your knees on the floor.

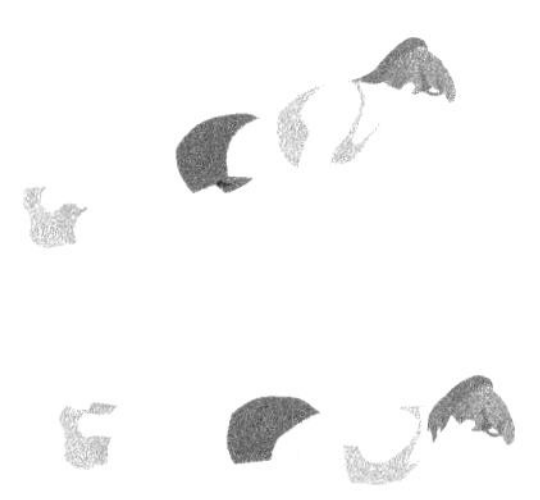

Crunches: Lie on the floor on your back, bend your knees and place your hands behind your head. Raise your torso towards your knees and lower back down.

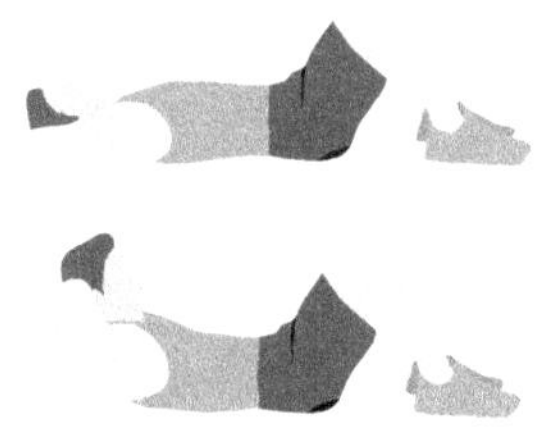

As you gain strength, you can increase the intensity and number of repetitions of the exercises for better results. Remember that this is just a primer to get you familiar with the types of exercises. There are multiple mobile apps or virtual workouts you can access that offer detailed routines and a huge variety of exercises.

REST AND RELAXATION FOR WELLNESS

Along with good nutrition and demanding training, rest and relaxation are just as important in maintaining a healthy lifestyle.

When we rest and relax, our body has the opportunity to recover and repair itself. Adequate rest helps us improve sleep quality, reduce stress and fatigue, and improve our concentration and mood. Incorporating moments of meditation, massage and relaxing activities such as reading a book or doing yoga, helps reduce stress and anxiety, and improve the quality of my sleep.

In theory, we are genetically designed to spend almost a third of our lives sleeping. This is not a negligible amount, but at least in today's society, quality sleep does not seem to be considered a priority.

Sleeping well is crucial for our body and mind, as it helps us recover and recharge our energy to face the next day. When we sleep, our body carries out cellular repair and regeneration processes, and also helps to consolidate memories and learning from the previous day. In addition, adequate sleep can improve our concentration, memory and mood, and help reduce stress and anxiety.

But it's not just the quantity of sleep that matters, it's also the quality. If you have trouble sleeping, your body can't do its nightly restorative work.

Getting a good night's sleep and meditating regularly are key to our physical and emotional well-being. But how can we improve sleep quality and establish a healthy sleep routine? Here are some tips:

Set a fixed bedtime and wake-up time: Try to maintain a consistent bedtime and wake-up time, even on weekends. This will help regulate your internal clock and improve the quality of your sleep.

Create a calm atmosphere: Make sure your room is comfortable, dark and quiet. Use blackout curtains, or even earplugs.

Avoid stimulation before bedtime: Turn off your electronic devices at least one hour before bedtime. The light from the screens interferes with the production of melatonin, the sleep hormone, because that light tells the brain that we are active and that we cannot let our guard down.

Exercise regularly: Regular exercise can help improve sleep quality. However, avoid exercising too close to bedtime, as it can have the opposite effect, especially if it is an exercise that pushes your heart rate to its maximum.

Practice relaxation techniques: Meditation, deep breathing and yoga can help reduce stress and anxiety, which in turn improves sleep quality.

Establish a consistent meditation practice: Dedicate a few minutes each day to meditation. You can start with just a few minutes and gradually increase the time. Meditation can help reduce anxiety, improve concentration and promote relaxation. Practicing meditation at different times of the day is a useful tool for mental rest. For meditating connects us with the absolute present, with our own body and puts us back to bed out of the turbulent tide of incessant thinking.

Inaugurate every day the moment of rest: Make a routine to close the day. Write down the pending tasks that you will solve the next day so you don't stay up at night ruminating about them. Then do a pre-rest ritual such as drinking a cup of chamomile tea, writing down the things you are grateful for, calling a loved one, reading a book. This will train the brain with the constant cue that problems will be thought about the next day, and not that we will let them grow, but that we will solve them after resting. When we cannot stop thinking about something it is because we feel guilty to postpone it for tomorrow, but insomnia full of worries rarely solves anything, it only leaves us exhausted to face the next day with the necessary energy and courage.

FINAL WORDS

We hope that reading this book has given you general tools to begin to see and feel your body differently, and to realize that taking care of it is the best way to be in life.

The road to a healthy life can be difficult and full of challenges, but with dedication, patience and perseverance, we can all achieve our physical, mental and spiritual goals. There is no magic formula or a single path to what everyone needs, everyone has to find their own path and walk it in their own way.

Perhaps the only valid general advice is not to give up. Sometimes things don't go as expected and we may feel discouraged, but every day is a new opportunity to move forward and do better. Focusing on personal goals, keeping a positive mind and surrounding yourself with supportive people is the best path to a healthier and more balanced life. You won't know the best version of you until you see it in front of the mirror and hear it in that voice in your head. What is it telling you right now?

If you liked this book, spread the word. Maybe someone needs it right now more than you do. Thank you.

For more tips, personalized advice and always up-to-date information, and motivational follow us here:

@TheWellnessFactoryPress

About The Wellness Factory

We are a publishing house whose mission is to spread the teaching of well-being as a human right... without pressure, without fashions, without stereotypes.

Another book for you:

Look At Yourself And Accept Who You Are

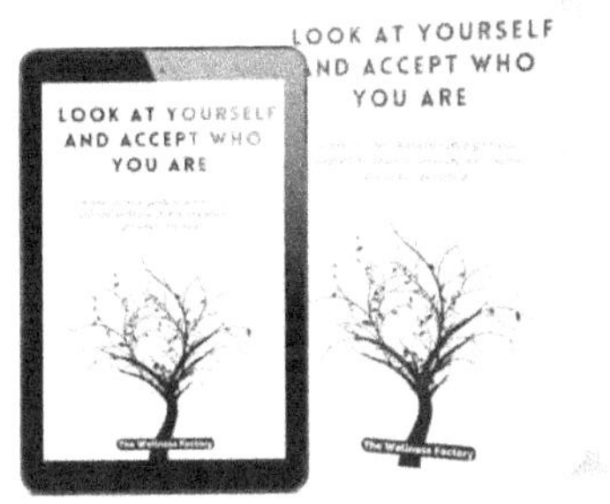